Table of Contents

The Importance of the Hamilton Anxiety Scale in Mental Health Assessment

Comprehensive Guide to the Hamilton Anxiety Scale (HAS)

1. Introduction to the Hamilton Anxiety Scale

If we understand the Hamilton Anxiety Scale, we will repeat the overall thinking and judgment of the assessment conducted with this scale, so that the quality of mental health care can be assured. Hamilton Anxiety Scale was first published in 1959. Over the past six decades, it has undergone two revisions in 1959 and 1960. The original version of the Hamilton Anxiety Scale was first described in a presentation by Hamilton on the pityriasis rosea treatment at a medication conference in 1958. It was developed through a control-group study of comprehensive anxiety neurosis treatment. It includes six subscales of the anxiety measurement, six of the somatic symptoms measurement, and eight of the clinician administration. It is usually finished by a clinical psychiatrist to measure treatment effect.

The Hamilton Anxiety Scale (HAS), first published in 1959, has become one of the most popular clinician-rated anxiety assessment tools. It was the result of a collaborative effort of several researchers, including Max Hamilton, who gave the scale his name. For about 60 years since its development, a large number of articles have been written to endorse or criticize the Hamilton Anxiety Scale. It is widely used in both psychiatric and non-psychiatric populations, and a version translated to an unspecified language has also been used to assess the anxiety condition of children and adolescents. The Hamilton Anxiety Scale for children and adolescents has also been developed and evaluated by psychometric properties. The Hamilton Anxiety Scale is used to determine the severity of anxiety symptoms and the recovery of anxiety.

1.1. Historical Background and Development

The original evidence base is as follows: nine outpatient clinic patients in psychiatric care referred to Hamilton from general practitioners, including patients who met the International Classification of Diseases 10th edition (ICD-10) for generalized anxiety and panic disorder. This sample was from general practice in Grimsby and London, England. Further patients with cancer ever referred to Hamilton were also studied. To calculate test-retest reliability, 18 relapse cases completed two ratings on the same day at nine hours' interval. Hamilton's friend and gentleman farmer completed the clinician-rated HAS of 15 consecutive female patients, though for the trial, while an unspecified reassessor completed the 12th and 13th. Scores were also calculated from the "original writing" of patients' "true feelings about their anxiety" from unselected clinic outpatients referred for differing treatment of chronic anxiety.

The Hamilton Anxiety Scale (HAS), published in 1959, was developed to assess the frequency of anxiety symptoms in patients diagnosed with anxiety neuroses. Hamilton proposed the following five symptoms: anxious mood and tension, fears, intellectual (cognitive) symptoms other than worry, somatic symptoms and general somatic complaints, and significant catastrophic thoughts. The 14-item scale started off as a clinician-report measure fitted for paper-and-pencil trials, but it has since expanded/adapted into either a self-rated or informant-based scale. Along with several other different versions, the original interview-scored scale has been translated and validated into numerous languages, with item reductions yielding trials with four items, 11 items, 13 items, and 15 items. The full 14-item version of the HAS is rated on a 20-point scale, with greater existing severity in symptoms warranting a higher score. To better follow the criterion-based scoring, 17 of the 21 symptoms therein have to be externally evident. Scores thus are totaled or weighted within the item surrounding a decision rule. Those ratings are computed after perusing the interview, querying the patient, and perusing the clinical history.

The Hamilton Anxiety Scale (HAS) is a supportive instrument, which is not compulsory. The HAS is largely recommended by its practicality in assigning target symptoms by clinicians; an approach that requires knowing which kind of a problem is being managed. It is mostly recommended for use in treating anxiety states and assessing the efficiency of pharmacotherapy, psychotherapies, and integrated therapies. The typical situations in which this manual is recommended include all anxiety disorders and those situations subjected to the development of an excessive fear and avoidance of phobic objects or situations. Because the HAS is based on symptoms, it can be recommended for all forms of anxiety and can provide useful information from organizing protocols for treatment by generalists who are familiar with the use of an instrument.

The Hamilton Anxiety Scale (HAS) is a specific tool to measure the complex clinical representation of anxiety, which is closely related to the patient's discomfort. This is why it is recommended for use in psychiatric settings during the evaluation of patients under similar treatments. Precisely, the HAS is intended for the use of clinicians, as it utilizes symptom quantification for explaining therapeutic results. However, this scale should not be employed to establish an anxiety diagnosis, to assess recent clinical outcome, to discern a particular mood subkind, as a discovery tool in exploration, or in non-pure/non-anxiety trials. This tool is essential for quantifying the level of unease or disorder. The result provides an index from 0 to 56. A weekly variation of 25% or a minimum departure of 3 is deemed essential. In general, scores from 0 to 8 show an absence of anxiety state, 9 to 18, mild to moderate, and 19 to 25, moderate to severe. Scores greater than 25 are associated with intense to very severe states of anxiety. In cases of depression in addition to an anxiety state, the consequent overall score needs to be interpreted with caution and it appears judicious to decide the ad hoc treatment based on score data.

2. Key Components of the Hamilton Anxiety Scale

1. Anxiety (psychic) - The wretched feeling or a frightened outlook (including the senses of depression, toughness, and poor, such as the presence of atypical complaints, trembling, fearfulness, fretful, self-doubt, anxiety) which does not occur regularly. 2. Anxiety (somatic) - Intolerable stress of the symptoms associated with the autonomic nervous system. 3. Anxiety (psychic) - Effects on tolerance, perception of stress, or between complaints of somatic anxiety disturbance and everyday matters. 4. Anxious Mood - The presence, and appearance, of anxious condition(s) affected on appearance when patients are dealing with peers, parents, or evaluators. 5. Tension - The presence of excessive, internal, or the inability to have a relaxed feeling or body area (facial expression, sleep, cognitive status) influenced. 6. Fears - The presence of comments to show the patient's rating of procedures, goals, aspects of nature, or environments, including appearing to have a crux (including the prospect of being attacked) set by the patient.

When designers administer or score the Hamilton Anxiety Scale, the goal is to evaluate the severity of a participant's anxiety symptoms. Each component of the scale is accompanied by a rating of 0 to 4, 0 to 3, or 0 to 2, with zero indicating no symptoms. There are 14 single-item components and four multi-item components - Tension, Anxious Mood, Intellectual, and Somatic symptoms. The

Generalized Anxiety Disorder Severity Scale (GADSS) heavily replicates the Hamilton Anxiety Scale when it comes to evaluating anxiety, which means developers can use the symptoms defined in the Hamilton Anxiety Scale to help complete the GADSS.

2.1. Anxiety Symptoms Assessed

Can anxious behavior lead others to label a person as "mentally ill"? If we follow this criterion, we should also take into account the often non-rational behavior of the anxious patient who causes stress on their family, is unable to fulfill their duties, and is not interested in or has severe problems concerning their hygiene. Basal signs of psychic-motor agitation influence the observer in the opposite way. Consequently, this particular item of the HAS helps to unify our evaluation of the patient. It is important to evaluate the current clinical condition and, in a longitudinal way, establish possible changes in the frequency and harshness of the "early" and "late" biological and psychological signs and symptoms to constantly update the risk of slipping. Thus, it is important to be able to use the HAS as a functional psychopathological tool in order for patients included in the studies to be phenotypically homogeneous.

Anxiety, as a general phenomenon, can be defined as an emotional reaction towards an actual or potential stressor. It is mostly observed in patients experiencing a high level of psychological distress or during the course of other severe mental disorders. The Hamilton Anxiety Scale (HAS) was specifically designed for the quantification and monitoring of this psychopathological condition. It includes ten items related to the present or past state of the subjects. The main issues regarding anxiety that are assessed with this instrument are the following: the harshness of the condition, which means the inherent physical and mental discomfort a subject experiences due to their anxiety; the type and source of the worries, which are the internal and external phenomena that evoke the patient's restlessness; the presence and frequency of psychosomatic and autonomic nervous system hyperfunctions related to the pathological condition; and the behavior of the anxious patient.

2.2. Scoring Criteria and Interpretation

For the purpose of this anxiety scale, the severity of the intensity caused by a different subjectivity was derived from both diagnosis and recommendation principles with a logical conclusion being reached with respect to the insufficient intensity. In an attempt to refine the existing reliability and validity coefficients, the findings did not reach the cutting scores because of their continuous constant that appeared to be adequate for both sensitivity and specificity of 100%. The suggested recommendations for the grading of scores and its interpretations are as follows. Any person with an overall score of 0 to 17 was rated as minimal, 18 to 24 as mild, 25 to 30 as moderate, and any score between 31 to 64 was rated as severe anxiety. For example, if patient scores are added up at the end of a test, a brief perception about the level of anxiety can be gauged. Given the vast advantages of this contemporary innovation, X-ray continues to soar, enabling both diagnosis and therapy to reach a diagnosis with speed and the most cost-effective/refined accuracy.

It is important to note that for every item that is marked as a "no", a score of zero (0) is obtained, and if the symptoms result in a severe impairment, a score of four (4) is assigned. The evaluation of the scoring criteria involves both cognitive and reflective processes in order to select the weighted score of b concerning the four responses that are anchored to the extreme side of the selected item as follows: 0 = no; 1 = mild; 2 = moderate; 3 = severe respectively.

3. Administration and Scoring Procedures

Severity Levels. The state following a HAM-A-administered session is to calculate severity level. "Mildly anxious" typically means a score well within the experienced norm, "moderately anxious" suggests that the score is well above the average anxiety experienced by others, and "severely anxious" means the patient is more anxious than most other anxious people.

Raw Scores. The raw score for the interviewer HAS is derived by summing the individual ratings in each item section in a two-step process.

Time of Administration. The scale was written to rate levels of anxiety over the past month, and hence standard instructions for HAS do not specify a particular time frame over which it is to be rated. However, as with all rating instruments geared to psychiatric or psychological states, the clinician must use some common sense and determine whether the patient has, in fact, been in a mental health care setting for the past month. If the patient is recently hospitalized or has just been sought out for anxiety treatment, then the past month question would seem unwarranted. As for the actual time of administration, there are no specifics in the published directions, and so far we know of no sources that have been developed using this. However, our common protocol is to score the State-Trait Anxiety Inventory (STAI) tests immediately after the patient has completed the Visual Analog Mood Scales (VAMS). The HAS is then administered.

Administration and Scoring Procedures. In general, the Hamilton scales are interview formats that are semi-structured. They are fairly close-ended, though an open questioning format is also provided. The interviewer is to form a judgment on the basis of the patient's verbal representation; observable behavior is also taken into account. The original instructions asked the interviewer to conduct the interview in the following sequence: "At the beginning, inquire about somatic symptoms and only after these are dealt with, should anxious or depressive symptoms be inquired into." The HAS is usually administered last in a battery assessing depression and/or other forms of psychopathology.

3.1. Standardized Administration Guidelines

Note 2: Regarding current time situations, ask the patient to specify fears according to day (morning, afternoon, evening), or hour in terms of day-time (8-12; 12-14; 14-17; afternoon (17-day + evening); 20-22).

Simply ask: "What are you most afraid of that could happen to you in general, meaning when you are doing your daily and leisure time activities? Are there any particular things/situations or will anything happen today or tomorrow that you are afraid of?".

If subjects say nothing more about fears or worries, the interviewer checks again, up to both day and night situations that are reflected in separated items. In general, items grouping reassures the subjects so that they can feel free to express their fears and worries. Handling of time units per question is a mere suggestion as usual, variants are allowed. The patient should not be penalized for his/her non-response, but encouraged instead to reflect upon the queried fear, or else, indifferent item scores are obtained by default.

Standardized administration is the key to obtaining assessments that are valid, reliable, and generally comparable across subjects and among research sites. In order to keep the interview format semi-structured, each step sequence is loaded with examples and instructions. Because every physician may ask about specific symptoms in a different manner, it is advised that his/her utterances are personalized to be comfortable for each one conducting an interview.

This direction, with little clinically useful detail, is consistent with contemporaneous psychiatric diagnostic interview guidelines widely used at that time. Since the publication of the Clinical Global Impressions rating scale in 1976, interview guides designed for structured or semi-structured HASTEN administration have been published.

The 1960 edition of the Hamilton Anxiety Scale (HAS) published administration guidelines as follows: "There should be as little noise and interruption from other staff and patients as possible during the administration and the choice of time of interview should be as appropriate as possible for the patient."

• 0-27: These represent the average scores for the general public and so would not indicate those who present as particularly anxious: some individuals will score higher and similarly some will score lower. 0-10: These scores represent those who may be lacking motivation and may have lost interest in aspects of life. Contrarily, these individuals may also be able to relax often and can focus on available activities. 11-20: These scores represent mild anxiety. They may be advantageous in certain situations. These individuals may be nervous about aspects of their lifestyle (work/social life, etc.) but this is not distressing enough to impede. They are not experiencing sustained feelings of tension. 21-30: These scores reflect moderate anxiety. They are beginning to experience some tension, frequent worries over things that have or may happen, regular fears for their health, ability to cope, etc. 31-50: These scores reflect severe anxiety. They will feel anxious most of the time and excessively preoccupied with particular worries, such as work, relationships, or finances. However, the anxiety will not reach the level where it overwhelms their coping strategies. 51-64: These scores represent the most severe forms of anxiety. This would be accompanied by an increased risk of panic attacks and also heightened symptoms such as dizziness, rapid heartbeat, and nausea. Additionally, they are likely to experience a range of physical complaints such as headache, neck pain, and aches.

As aforementioned, the HAS was originally developed to measure the severity of anxiety symptoms in the moment. The following are recommended interpretative cutoffs for time of use/administration. Each item is rated from 0 (absent) to four (severe). Summing the scores of each item on the scale will yield a severity level. These represent the interpretation of the scores in the clinical evaluation of anxiety states.

Interpreting Scores and Severity Levels

4. Reliability and Validity of the Hamilton Anxiety Scale

Nishith and Yehuda reported that the HAM-A demonstrated high internal consistency in the Khmer community-based sample. Cronbach's alpha was 0.75 for Sample 1 (n = 137) and 0.86 for Sample 2 (n = 57). The HAM-A was significantly associated with the AHorror ASD and PTSD symptoms and demonstrated comparable predictive accuracy to the HADS anxiety subscale. In the best fitting model, the internal hierarchy of HAM-A symptoms began progressively with anxious mood as the least severe, followed by the psychic factor scale (i.e. mental agitation, hypervigilance, fears), and finally the somatic factor scale that included gastrointestinal, genitourinary, respiratory, autonomic, musculoskeletal, and other somatic symptoms of anxiety. Taken together, evidence suggests that the HAM-A is a useful tool for the measurement of anxiety. This conclusion is based on a relatively large number of studies (k = 6), drawing on sizeable Random Number Generators (standard population sample), and epidemiologically Best Fit sample.

The following section reviews the reliability, internal structure, validity, and clinical utility evidence for the Hamilton Anxiety Scale (HAS). It also compares HAS to other commonly used anxiety scales. Evidence for the psychometric properties of HAS is summarized in Tables 4-8. Several studies report the psychometric properties of the Hamilton Anxiety Scale (HAM-A) and give details of the recruitment sample and statistical procedures. This includes evaluating the factorial structure, internal consistency, concurrent validity, and discriminatory power. In total, six studies reported the psychometric properties of the Hamilton Anxiety Scale (HAM-A). One study was located through a manual search of the bibliographical list, another through a systematic search of PubMed and Google.

4.1. Research Studies and Findings

The current evidence suggests that the Hamilton Anxiety Scale (HAS) mainly measures a general factor to identify the presence of anxiety disorders in adult samples, expressed with symptoms such as anxious mood or tension. In addition to this general component, the scale would measure factors related to different anxiety disorder symptoms, including those focused on the cognitive or psychic symptoms of the disorders, such as fears and worries. We agree with Mataix-Cols and colleagues that the suitability of using multi-item measures for diagnostic purposes needs to be further studied. Research on the reliability and validity of the proposed artificial intelligence-generated diagnostic criterion for agoraphobia is established using other research approaches. The empirical evidence obtained with the Hamilton Anxiety Scale supports its validity as an instrument to evaluate anxiety, monitor its level during treatments, and identify its presence in individuals with various medical and psychological clinical conditions. The Hamilton Anxiety Scale has shown excellent internal consistency and significant patient-clinician correlations.

Colón de Martí studied a sample containing 482 adults from the community and individuals diagnosed with anxiety disorders seeking psychological assistance. The results supported a 6-factor structure, although several items had to be removed from the original version of the scale. Orive et al. also agreed with a 6-factor model in a sample of 222 people diagnosed with an anxiety or somatization disorder seeking psychological care. Leal et al. argued in favor of a 6-factor structure in a sample of 222 people diagnosed with affective disorders, anxiety disorders, or somatoform disorders currently undergoing psychological treatment. Nitschke et al. carried out the most recent study, supporting an 8-factor solution in a sample of 118 adults diagnosed with anxiety disorders seeking psychological assistance.

The factorial structure of the Hamilton Anxiety Scale (HAS) has been analyzed by several research teams. Based on these research studies, the factorial structure of the Hamilton Anxiety Scale (HAS) is predominantly supported by this scientific evidence. The scale consists of a general anxiety disorder factor and several anxiety- or symptom-specific factors, as explained in the introduction.

A number of scales used in the study of anxiety have been elaborated by various authors. The Beck Anxiety Inventory (BAI) is a 21-point scale primarily designed to measure anxiety symptom severity in adults and adolescents. It was developed to avoid "overlap with some of the somatic items of the Beck Depression Inventory" and also to monitor for frequent comorbidity of anxiety and depression. The BAI, however, is limited in its use for evaluating the severity of symptoms of anxiety as it was not constructed with this purpose in mind. Additionally, the scale lacks a clear definition of anxiety. Researchers emphasize two major limitations of the BAI, particularly the high overlap of symptoms with depressive patients, and also the existence of only somatic items. The State-Trait Anxiety Inventory (STAI) is designed for use by adults and younger individuals over the age of 12.

Comparison with Other Anxiety Assessment Tools

The HAS is a useful and comprehensively validated scale for the assessment of anxiety symptoms in terms of severity. Table 4 depicts the main advantages and disadvantages of the HAS as perceived by various authors. While these assessments are often subjective or not supported by the authors' research data, they nevertheless represent a valuable source of information regarding HAS to a potential user. In order to understand the possible usage of the HAS in research, we must compare it to other measurements administered for a similar purpose. In the next part of the introduction, we will provide a summary of some other frequently employed anxiety scales, including their potential usages in terms of the basic requirement for a research instrument.

5. Clinical Applications and Populations

The instrument has been successfully used across the life span, and there is a separate Hamilton Anxiety Rating Scale for children and adolescents that assesses psychosomatic features more commonly seen in this age group. Therefore, the scale is also appropriate for use with a variety of age groups, from children to adults. However, for individuals who are hearing impaired or do not speak English, the HAS would not be appropriate. Although it is available in several languages, the psychometric properties for these different translations have not been established. Additionally, the scale may not be appropriate for all cultural groups if differing views on anxiety in certain cultural groups make the questions irrelevant. There are also no data on the usefulness of the scale with individuals with severe cognitive disability due to mental retardation or organic problems because the scale has not been assessed with these groups. Used in a variety of settings and patient populations, the diverse uses to which the HAS has been put attest to its utility as an anxiety assessment instrument.

The Hamilton Anxiety Scale can be used in a variety of clinical settings where problems with anxiety are seen. The HAS is useful in a number of different psychiatric populations, including inpatient and outpatient samples. It has been used to differentiate different anxiety disorders and assess clinical improvement in anxiety disorders. It is also used to monitor the success of pharmacological treatment in persons with anxiety. The scale may also have application in assessing anxiety in various medical populations; studies have used the HAS to study patients with medical disorders such as hyperthyroidism, Parkinson's Disease, and mitral valve prolapse. Therefore, the HAS can be used with patients in a variety of clinical settings, including primary care, general and psychiatric hospitals, and psychiatric and medical outpatient clinics.

5.1. Use in Different Clinical Settings

Keys to the use of HAS and helpful assessments are the following: Thus, the HAS is versatile to be employed and reported comparing subjects using specific diagnoses; the scale is used for assessing the effectiveness including or beyond existing psychopharmacological agents, most commonly benzodiazepines, but the differences in findings on the scale are mixed in between the benzodiazepines and relevant medications subclasses; the scale is used for assessing the disorder severity or psychometric properties; the lack of group differences and correlation for the scale is used for the criterion-related validity for some medications and diagnoses. Also, the scale lacks statistical administration-subjects mental and physical comorbidity associations at baseline evaluations.

The HAS is mostly administered in hospital outpatient settings of general hospitals and psychiatry clinics, either in general internal medicine units or in emergency room/emergency departments. Given the versatility of the scale or the many types of cross-comparative studies, total scores on the HAS are used as the disorder outcomes or independent variables of statistical significance in regression analyses, or continuous in nature or clinimetric in scope. The scale is used for observational and epidemiological studies, comparing committee consensus diagnoses with the baseline diagnostic assessments/screening evaluation during a long-term follow-up and natural history of alcoholism in clinical outpatient setting.

5.2. Applicability to Various Age Groups

Age is of real significance in examining symptoms of anxiety. Anxiety symptoms from young adulthood up to old age may have certain characteristics determined by the developmental phase (e.g., educational or work phase, the beginning or the end of a career) as well as by having one family (e.g., the developmental phase of rearing children). Thus, anxiety symptoms are related to life satisfaction (which diminishes with surprise to reach the lowest level at mid-life crisis at about age 40) and accordingly, a perhaps typical expression of anxiety for a particular phase in life might get overshadowed by the general 'neurotic' expression of anxiety. Assumedly, if one would develop specific age-applicable anxiety scales, one would find compliance scores for typical or normal levels of anxiety in different ages.

Although the aforementioned research doesn't provide information about the applicability of the original HAS for older adults, some symbols also have applicability to the assessment and analysis of older adults. Older adults also show higher levels of basic traits like neuroticism as well as social anxiety, if not more, so these traits, of course, involve anxiety symptoms with a certain relevance for this population. Moreover, an important factor in examining older adults with anxiety problems can be to consider possible accompanying medical health care obstacles. These two elderly applicable symptoms suggest that the HAS is also applicable to research with older adults.

2) In 1997, a short version of the HAS consisting of 9 items was constructed and tested for replicability. This version, mainly meant for use in adolescent and student research in the 14-20 age group, mainly proved to be a reliable and valid research instrument. At present, a validated short version of the HAS, as adapted for the general adult population, is not yet available.

1) In 1990, a short version of Kohl's HAS consisting of 9 items was constructed and tested for replicability. This version, mainly meant for use in child research up to puberty, also proved to be a reliable and valid research instrument. Concerning this shortened HAS, which child research version is adapted for the age group between 14 and 20 years will shortly be available from the author. A complementary child version to the HAS, though, adapted for children younger than age 14, is unfortunately lacking.

Clinical studies showed that the HAS represents an appropriate tool for the age groups of children, adolescents, and adults.

6. Advantages and Limitations of the Hamilton Anxiety Scale

Until we can formulate a more robust number, appraisers will have to use their own clinical judgment to determine when the results accurately point to a diagnosis and just what severity. Simply utilizing the HAS alone continues to leave assessment open to inaccuracies due to comorbid depression with a 99% chance for false positives. Routine use of the HARS scale on people who have significant physical symptoms of anxiety might benefit from some physical health assessment, this is where the importance of a structured interview including an in-depth psychosocial can offer much more in terms of clinician finding the primary depression vs clinical anxiety disorder. Would a mild to moderate social anxiety patient perceive these treatment plans side by side differently by completing this more eating or by endorsing "Trichotillomania" with the good to the question: "Do you experience significant hair and includes 105 item questions. In order for a patient to aid in the diagnostic and therapeutic process, a physician has to spend anywhere from 40 to 60 minutes—in one setting—conducting the full patient interview. While diagnostic thresholds are easier to find for a more complete scale, the automated way to determine if a patient needs further assessment without any judgment after two weeks. For some patients, the time taken and extra $100 billing might be inappropriate if a zung or phq patient scored significantly lower initially. There has not been a percentile metric produced from inpatient data yet.

Limitations of the HAS

When compared with the other anxiety scales in use, the HAS exhibits good to excellent internal consistency and runs the least risk of overdiagnosis. The clear scoring benchmarks and structure of the HAS make it easy for a discussion between appraiser and patient about what their anxiety points look like and where the most significant risk is encountered. The easy-to-understand HAS tool gives the evaluator the chance to consult with the patient to determine the most relevant areas to be focused on for a specific care. Additionally, a short comorbid depression scale might be strategically placed in front of the HAS to help quickly determine if complimentary treatment would be prudent to address underlying depression. The logistic benefits of being able to be used as a data collection tool as well as a clinical assessment tool brings in a flexibility that is lacking in many other anxiety measures. Before the world of program evaluation came of age, the HARS was being used as the go-to gold standard research tool. The research community values the ability to measure anxiety over time or particular circumstances in a comparison sample. The HAS and HAS-M are one of the easiest scales to take to scale. The popular HAS scale is already available to patients in 22 languages.

Advantages of the HAS

6.1. Benefits of Using HAS

In this sense, one of the major benefits of HAS is that its use has been recommended in many clinical guidelines to enable a comprehensive assessment of anxiety, including common symptomatological manifestations (psychic and somatic symptoms) and disability associated with anxiety disorders, allowing more informed decision-making. One possible reason for this is the great body of existing research; more factors are significantly known to be associated with Hamilton Anxiety Scale scores (i.e., severity, diagnosis, functionality, psychosis, poor prognosis severity, coping style). Likewise, one of the most important advantages that the scale offers is that it has exhibited good psychometric properties, such as internal consistency, test-retest reliability, content validity, and content structure. The HAS also has shown significant correlations with other frequently used anxiety scales, such as the HADS or the STAI. Additionally, along with the benefit of being free to use, it has low user burden. Consequently, the HAS has potentially become a valid option to monitor and evaluate anxiety disorders, especially in countries where HADS or STAI have not been validated yet.

This last decade has witnessed a substantial rise in the relevance of measuring anxiety symptoms, especially in individuals with physical or mental conditions. In this context, the Hamilton Anxiety Scale (HAS) has become one of the most prominent and widely used scales for assessing anxiety. Proof of this is that the original version has been cited more than 1500 times in the last five years. One possible reason supporting its success could be that clinicians value HAS because of its well-known strength and qualities.

6.2. Potential Drawbacks and Considerations

The choice of a gold standard for a whole syndrome such as anxiety neurosis when considering the construct validity of the HAS can never be capable of anything more than inferring some elements of content validity. Limited information is available on the convergent or established validity of the HAS in patients attending mental health services; that is, evidence that the HAS successfully discriminated between successive and overlapping diagnostic categories of anxious patients would also assist in making general statements about reliability and validity. As the HAS data in community samples still remain exploratory, this weakens our ability to consolidate the value of these data with respect to evaluating the scale's content, predictive or divergent validity. Similarly, additional research is recommended when properties such as test-retest reliability, minimal important difference, sensitivity to change and optimal cut-off scores, are needed in light of the potentially large uptake of the HAS for health research purposes. Given the good internal consistency of the HAS summed score, other available measures of multimorbidity might complement the HAS in epidemiological surveys.

The length of the Hamilton Anxiety Scale (HAS) and the relative complexity of items that ask individuals to weigh different aspects of anxiety may perhaps limit its wide use in routine clinical evaluation and general patient screening. In addition, although the HAS provides an overall measure of anxious affect, it is quite detailed with respect to the physical symptoms of anxiety compared to questions regarding internalized worry or nervousness. One exception to this is that the scale is designed to ensure that irritability (seen more prominently in the younger anxious patient) is considered, which is lacking in broad instruments, such as the General Health Questionnaire. Clinical evaluation is further well served if the HAS communication item is considered important, as clinic non-attendance and poor relationship with healthcare professionals can result when it is negative.

7. Future Directions and Innovations in Anxiety Assessment

Future directions for this line of work include using treatment outcome data to identify status markers, symptom-specific, and general markers, predictive potentials for chronic inflammation and prolonged immune response, using non-treatment-seeking groups and those with subclinical anxiety, a broader anxiety disorder group to improve external validity, and different methods of medication administration, also to improve generalizability to the broader population. Rapidly developing technological advancements have created numerous opportunities for computerized, electronic, and mobile assessment methods. Such tools are increasingly being applied to account for increasing social discomfort with pen-and-paper psychological assessment, budgetary restrictions, and to accommodate large-scale research efforts. It is suggested that computerized and mobile assessment methods are also an avenue for anxiety assessment.

With the burgeoning interest in the field of anxiety relatively recently, a number of changes and areas of growth can be anticipated in the field of anxiety assessment. As a field, it is hoped that the utility and innovation of using other methods of mental health assessment, such as the phonological blood flow symmetries of qEEG topography used by Putman and her colleagues in this issue, can be incorporated into anxiety assessment tools. One of those methods, event-related potentials (ERPs), has been found to predict SSRI response, and the most effective cue type for identifying those with generalized anxiety disorder and generalized social anxiety disorder. The most effective cue type for identifying efficient between-group differences (those with generalized anxiety disorder or generalized social anxiety disorder vs. no psychopathology), the anterior shift seen in post-treatment ERP effects might be indicative of the mechanism through which anxiety is reduced via successful treatment, and several potentials are discussed that might have clinically useful predictive properties.

7.1. Emerging Trends in Anxiety Measurement

The area of anxiety assessment continues to evolve and develop. As anxiety may be a more diffuse and fluctuating affective state than depression, a frequent goal has been to develop new methodologies for assessing state anxiety. In the present volume, we describe new behavioral, psychophysiological, and neuroscience-based methodologies for the assessment of state anxiety that may be especially relevant to assessing anxiety subtypes or transdiagnostic features that overlap with other affective diagnoses. At the same time, there is a resurgence of interest in transdiagnostic self-report scales for depression and anxiety and how self-report scales with anxiety items perform across diverse populations. The future of anxiety assessment may rely on a combination of emerging neuroscience-based technologies, new metrics for identifying dimensions of psychological functioning, and self-report scales that can be applied across the lifespan and in different cultures.

This section of the book has attempted to provide a comprehensive guide of the Hamilton Anxiety Scale (HAS) and provides practical and conceptual detail about each item of the scale that should be useful to researchers. As this book was being prepared, we also identified potentially influential changes in how anxiety is measured. As a snapshot, some of the research discussed in this section has not received a large number of citations and we cannot predict the field's reaction to them, but we believe that they are indicative of how the field is changing.

7.2. Technological Advancements in Assessment Tools

For the accurate assessment of anxiety, it is crucial to measure and make a combination of 'objective Scales' with techniques 'heart rate' and EDA i.e. Electro-Dermal Activity. In the last, we would like to mention the significance of New Research Efforts as a final heading (7.2.1). Under this is also described Knowledge Answers (fact analysis stage) as well as Comprehension Answers (conceptual integration stage) for different purposes of assessment individually. New research vigour would be believed using the analysis of 'Practical Skills and Holistic Learning', which requires a set of thought and emotion.

Focusing on technological advancements in the context of assessment, we have developed some tools and techniques for better assessment of evitable level of anxiety in patients either transferring to new environment or physical pain. Westin and Finset examined physiologic arousal releases due to pain as a hidden barrier of personal communication. Lautenmacher et al. observed that activation of central autonomic network is linked with anxiety and pain. Sreenivasa and Singh used impedance cardiography which measures output from the heart as cardiac output and it was used to predict anxiety and pain of patient simultaneously (height anxiety and Δ height anxiety). Saule studied the pledge of treatment and later his study provided enhancement of power of individual to self-report. For detailed discussion of Self-Reported Scales for Anxiety consult Chapter 7.

The Importance of the Hamilton Anxiety Scale in Mental Health Assessment

1. Introduction to the Hamilton Anxiety Scale

Through standardized anxiety and medication ratings, the World Health Organization has placed specific emphasis on identifying the developmental facets of controversial adjuvant treatments such as benzodiazepines. Sustained fears, somatic concerns, and motor tension are the three Hamilton subscales being investigated for current SP/SOC phenotypes under a 10-foot paradigm (HAM-A). Racine verbal HAM-A summaries from 130 controls and 126 individuals with SP/SOC arthritis are contrasted using t-test testing. Personal score Pearson connection examinations were also performed to determine intrinsic multivariate relationships.

The Hamilton Anxiety Scale (HAM-A) is an assessment tool used to evaluate anxiety and measure the severity and extent of its manifestations. It is often used in clinical settings to identify anxiety-related symptoms and has demonstrated the utility of measuring anxiety to researchers in controlled environments. The extensive range of experiences elicited from people with anxiety is acknowledged in the scale's 14 areas, which include all five of the DSM's anxiety category symptoms: physical complaints, cognitive disturbances, sleep problems, irritability, and anxious mood. Regardless of the particular domain, endorsing just one component in any HAM-A subcategory results in a score of one for that subscale, making the measure highly sensitive to both symptom magnitude and variety. In this sense, the HAM-A is both a measure of anxiety quantity and a measure of anxiety variety, which is to say it assesses the breadth of anxiety symptoms someone is experiencing. Given these distinct advantages over single symptoms or global measures, the HAM-A continues to be a popular standardized approach.

2. Development and Purpose of the Scale

The Hamilton Anxiety Scale (HAM-A) was built for anxiety assessment and has been available for over 60 years. It attracts a full range of anxiety disorder symptoms, and it is also helpful in detecting current and future comorbid mood disorder symptom states, and provides general laboratory guideline checklists for those with other anxiety disorders. Because of the specificity of the goals and the contemporary misleading areas of laboratory assessments, the scale is always short. It is not necessary to evaluate anxiety as a continuum except where the symptoms may be a continuous variable; instead, it is best understood as an 'all or nothing' phenomenon. The checklist chosen for the scale was taken from multiple sources and all items have been created in order to check for current and future status.

The first Hamilton Anxiety Scale, now known as the Hamilton Anxiety Scale (HAM-A), was developed as a modernized rating scale for the measurement of anxiety prevalence. The face-to-face psychiatric interview was generally chosen as the format for the scale, while it was also found to be reliable in clinical research. Several syndromes, particularly anxiety and depression, were to be better understood and identified so as to recognize the response to therapy, so an anxiety scale was created for this specific purpose. Lobban (2004) argued that the scale was at the cutting edge of its time and gives information similar to that found in modern-day scales on the same issues. The organization wanted a test to be carried out promptly, so the scale was observed for a week, but most studies (> 7 days) evaluate it over a two-week period. As for the development era of the scale, some items involved in creating the 14-item HAM-A were collected randomly by the psychiatrist from interviews and studies undertaken at the time.

3. Components of the Hamilton Anxiety Scale

The HAM-A also includes other features that make it especially valuable. There are clear, specifically described criteria for scoring the HAM-A items. There are also clear instructions on whether to score items. All of the items on the HAM-A are scored either using explicitly described means or plain observation. This includes items that capture some of the clinical severity often seen in the assessment of GAD (e.g., severe and consistent difficulties in falling or staying asleep) and the extra hallucinations measure that clinicians feel ought to belong in a depression severity scale (e.g., item 9 is a useful reminder that anxiety is often combined with feelings of sadness and, provided the anxiety disorder is also rated, will provide an assessment of excessive sadness).

The first six items include anxious mood (such as tension and fears), general somatic symptoms (such as muscular, sensory, and cardiovascular symptoms), general psychiatric symptoms (such as feelings of derealization and depersonalization) and genitourinary symptoms— although these are not always seen in Western anxiety patients. The next six items include the assessment of different types of phobias (e.g., to crowds or leaving the house), non-fearsome symptoms (e.g., gastrointestinal and behavior at interview) and subjective, tension-related symptoms like difficulty falling and staying asleep. In the remaining two items, the HAM-A measures the severe mental and bodily symptoms often found in severe anxiety and accompanying depression such as clear, sensory based hallucinations, but also depression with anxiety symptoms. In other words, the HAM-A includes assessments of symptoms that may be related to generalized anxiety disorder (GAD), but are also a useful reminder that our concept of GAD is not as culturally neutral and as "pure" as it is sometimes theorized or portrayed.

The 14-item Hamilton Anxiety Scale (HAM-A) is one of the most widely used and accepted instruments in mental health assessments, including in clinical trials. There are several components of the HAM-A that make it a valuable tool. The HAM-A was designed to not just capture a picture of general anxiety, but to be as comprehensive as possible. Consequently, there are many different aspects of anxiety measured in the HAM-A. This is already evident from the symptoms it assesses.

3.1. Anxiety Symptoms Assessed

Anxious mood (fears), 4 items, scored between 0 to 4 points. This category focuses on assessing anxious feelings resulting from nervous tension, impairing the individual in leading a normal life. Tension, the only item in this category, reflects stress or anxiety resulting from difficulty in relaxing either mentally or physically irrespective of the cause, with a score of 0 to 4 points. This category examines the variety of fears that the patient has or generates, rather than the degree of anxiety directly associated with such fears. Insomnia, one of the most common symptoms in mental illness, is distributed according to its severity from difficulty in falling asleep to frequent night waking. According to this HAM-A provision, medical examination may be necessary to accurately categorize the cause of insomnia. The next three categories, like all of the HAM-A categories are linear, with scores of 0 through 4.

As per the current protocol of the guidelines for its use, the total assessment is composed of 14 items evaluating the following categories: 1) Anxious mood (fears); 2) Tension; 3) Fears; 4) Insomnia; 5) Intellectual; 6) Depressed mood; 7) Somatic (muscular); 8) Somatic (sensory); 9) Cardiovascular symptoms; 10) Respiratory symptoms; 11) Autonomic symptoms gastrointestinal; 12) Genitourinary autonomic symptoms; 13) Most of the physical aspects; 14) Behavior (appearances observed). The symptoms scored can be identified in the Supplementary Material.

3.2. Scoring Criteria

A moderately severe score is a three (3) according to the manual which includes points 3 and 2. All twenty-one items included in the HAM-A are scored, yielding best possible scores of no anxiety (0) and most severe anxiety (56). The scoring is broken down as: 0 = not present; 1 = mild; 2 = moderate; 3 = severe; and 4 = very severe. This quantitative assessment approach provides a more definitive standard by which to rate the severity or absence of a given anxiety symptom. The summed total thus yields a patient's severity score but does not specify the presence of comorbid anxiety disorders like panic disorder or PTSD. Additionally, based on the manual, the Somnolence and Intellectual Factors subscales require an additional 9 items listed under "out" to score either beyond the generally listed 5 levels. These factors correspond to serotonergic (5HT) and norepinephrine reuptake inhibiting (NERI) drugs less leading to fatigue and sleep or to sedation and better representing the sedative hypnotic spectrum.

Each symptom in the HAM-A is scored on a five-point scale based on their parameters or guidelines. The HAM-A was specifically developed in adults to address the somatic symptoms frequently used in making a differential diagnosis in sex, age, and retirement status-related anxiety occurring in the presence of depression. Each subscale item was thus based on the specific anxieties like depressed mood, feelings of guilt or worthlessness, early insomnia, late insomnia, middle insomnia, work and activities, suicide, retardation, agitation, and psychic anxiety.

4. Administration and Scoring Procedures

This chapter describes the administration and scoring procedures for the HAM-A for reliable and valid measurements to be obtained. Administration procedures are explained, and it is noted that documentation of general atmosphere, volume and tone of conversation, rapport, characteristics of the patient and any parameters which may invalidate the results of HAM-A should be documented in addition to the individual items. Practical considerations should be considered to ensure that the assessment will provide consistent and accurate results. Characteristics such as impaired hearing, history of transient ischemic attacks, have readings below 70/50 mm of Hg, frequent bleeding or clotting and dysreflexia might affect valid and reliable scoring. Administering the HAM-A usually takes 10-15 min and is evaluated twice yearly. The items and interview guides for scoring are presented and described in this chapter.

The Hamilton Anxiety Scale (HAM-A) is one of the oldest and most widely used rating scales of severity for the evaluation of symptoms of anxiety. The scale consists of 14 items, each defined by a series of symptoms, and measures both psychic anxiety (mental agitation and psychological distress) and somatic anxiety (physical complaints related to anxiety or features of autonomic arousal). Assessment of HAM-A involves considering the frequency, duration, severity, and the degree of distress associated with anxiety.

The scale has demonstrated good clinimetric properties when examining severity and change over time and has been recommended for routine use in adult and elderly patient samples in numerous clinical guidelines.

5. Interpretation of Results

Severe Anxiety: In the 23 to 30 range. Many fears - mental incapacitation, can't function in any significant way, dreading doing things that the situations it fear provokes. Complicating this would be the fact that the interviewee may also report somatic symptoms.

Moderate Anxiety: In the 15 to 22 range. Full syndromal anxiety and beginning to become disabled by worry, apprehension, and the physical effects. The person would avoid some situations or objects - hard to carry out ordinary activities and responsibilities.

Mild Anxiety: In the 8 to 14 range. You would have trouble and be uncomfortable, but you would probably still be able to function in the situation. Subthreshold for the severity level of anxiety and not considered "disabling."

0-7: No anxiety. No clinical intervention. People might seek treatment but do not meet criteria or are subthresholds. Very few people will score this low, maybe a few questions or one area. Many systems would just not count these as it could be that just one question would score this low. Most just ask the 14 that are considered the best indicators.

Determination and estimation of the implications of anxiety based on scores

The Hamilton Anxiety Scale and the importance of finishing the original assumptions

- Mild: The individual shows some mild somatic complaints but with minimal effect on functioning, is alert and oriented, and says symptoms are bothersome but not incapacitating. (Score: 0-17) - Moderate: Symptoms tend to occur with more frequency and intensity. Patients often manifest some evidence of distress and are sometimes seen by others as overly anxious. The disorder causes moderate social and/or occupational disability. (Score: 18-24) - Severe: Many or most symptoms will be of moderate to severe intensity and performing without fear of failure becomes a marked difficulty. The sense of despair leads to hopelessness and suicidal thoughts can be present. The disorder causes severe social and/or occupational disability and needs more help with everyday tasks. (Score: 25-30) - Very severe: A marked reduction in the ability to function due to mental preoccupation. The anxiety colors and disrupts most conversations, including office examinations. (Score: 31 and over)

Severity levels are characterized according to the score obtained on HAM-A:

5.2. Clinical Implications

Elevations of HAM-A score were a risk factor loss of response amongst duloxetine responders. The citalopram exploratory analysis allows us to observe relapse patterns in both the duloxetine (if withdrawn) and citalopram (regardless of duloxetine) treatment arms. Comparing relapse rates in the exploratory citalopram study (after placebo withdrawal) with baseline analyses (placebo controlled citalopram treatment at week 24 in the duloxetine citalopram study) suggests that discontinuing active treatment is associated with some relapses which were unrelated to the subjects' history of previous duloxetine treatment. Since the HAM-A relapse rates did increase after discontinuing active treatment, these may suggest spontaneous relapses in the absence of the treatment practice effect in the active treatment continuation phase study.

The results of the dosing study - showing that doses of pregabalin are most effective in the range 150mg/daily to 600mg/daily - maps across well with the dosing range seen in 8 controlled trials published in the literature with this medication using the categorical CGI diagnostic result to determine who should proceed in a one day, placebo controlled discontinuation study. Pregabalin is a useful medication in the treatment of SAD symptoms. However, given its side effect profile and US restrictions in some practices, it would be prudent to apply the general principle of monotherapy to treatment. Patients who fail to

have an adequate response at 150mg/daily are more likely
to have an inadequate response at higher doses.

6. Reliability and Validity of the Scale

Out of 14 items, "anxious mood," "tension," and "fears" are related to subjective problems. Although "intellectual," "somatic muscular," "cardiovascular," "respiratory," and "gastrointestinal" are related to somatic problems, as the items increase, somatization increases. It is difficult to instantly measure the issue like "sensory" in number and percentage. However, the mean and standard deviation of the item with a score of 56 points is important. Until now, the basic quality of the property of a diagnostic and research tool could be identified as credibility. It is possible to determine the reliability of a scale by finding out whether the items on the same scale reflect the same values in the coefficient correlation found by using Pearson or Spearman rank coefficient correlation. The range of validity is the ability of a scale to measure the factor it believed to measure. The HAM-A 14-item scale elements measure the consensus of clinicians as perceptions in the direction of one factor. Thus, by proving the reliability and validity of the scale, it was determined that HAM-A is a very valuable scale to be used in both diagnosing anxiety problems and determining the outcomes of the study.

Reliability and validity are important to make tools proper for use. The Hamilton Anxiety Scale (HAM-A) is based on the earlier ones and evaluates anxiety. This scale ranges between 0-56 points and symptoms are assessed between 14 items with a 5-point scale. The detailed content provides both making it suitable for use in clinical settings and the most basic quality to be a valuable tool in the fight against diseases, to be applied to the experimental group as homogenous as possible in research. HAM-A was applied to 108 schizophrenic patients, 114 obsessive-compulsive disorder (OCD) patients and 135 healthy controls for reliability.

7. Clinical Applications

The HAM-A has accordingly been applied in studies to address the taxometric challenges of anxiety and comorbid mood and anxiety disorders—practical clinical applications of these methods that might not otherwise be possible. Emerging evidence suggests a confluence of anxiety due to depressed mood, child-mother patterns that differentiate anxious and inhibited temperament, hair cortisol and its associations with somatic symptoms, audible biology and anxious interference, and the etiology of anhedonia. The HAM-A and its factors demonstrate long-term stability, historical continuity, cross-regional replication, and rapid response to treatments. As a further widespread application, the HAM-A has been used as an index of panic state, particularly at the start of active treatment, because anxiety is a primary feature of panic.

The Hamilton Anxiety Scale (HAM-A) allows for an extensive assessment of anxious affect, somatic symptoms, and feelings of tension in clinically anxious populations. It enables the psychiatrist, clinical psychologist, or clinician in primary care to make a diagnosis, develop a treatment plan, and monitor treatment effects across a wide variety of disorders. Anxiety and its comorbid conditions are highly prevalent, debilitating, and costly, and HAM-A subscales and questions are relevant to the heterogeneity of symptoms that can accompany an anxiety disorder. Data from the HAM-A can aid measurement-based stepwise and sequential approaches to the treatment of patients with anxiety and related states.

7.1. Diagnosis and Treatment Planning

The HAM-A can also be used in a formulation or treatment planning strategy. In tracking what anxiety symptoms are moderate to high or high and in using this information to make formulations of treatment candidates, a "categorical" treatment strategy (i.e. Social Anxiety Disorder versus Obsessive-Compulsive Disorder; Generalized Anxiety Disorder versus dysthymia) might be made. In short, the HAM-A often provides information that is critical to further treatment planning. In measuring the HAM-A early in treatment and repeatedly thereafter, the scale yields vital information that is critical to selecting appropriate medications and dosages (as it ascertains severity of anxiety and can be used to assess treatment response) and in coping with the complex effects of using adjunctive treatments in treatment resistance or therapy recidivism. Plan the goal of therapy by noting HAM-A items with high scores despite treatment. If the Health/Anxiety Awareness/Terror of the HAM-A questionnaire are still "pretty high" after treatment begins while mental sedation goes down, the subject's anxiety may still be a potent determinant of therapy's objective. Therapy would be re-evaluated as anxiety has still been endorsed as an important area to improve.

7.1. Diagnosis and Treatment Planning. The HAM-A is frequently used to document current and pretreatment levels of subjectively experienced anxiety, as well as to indicate if an individual has subjectively elevated levels of anxiety regardless of the designation of their anxiety-related disorder. Because the HAM-A assays subjective experience of anxiety, it does not provide a "cut off" for the presence of anxiety. Further, the HAM-A can be used to clarify the etiology of an individual's anxiety disorder. For example, if a subject's profile of anxiety levels on the HAM-A illustrates notable elevations on HAM-A items querying mood-related anxiety, an appropriate diagnosis could be Generalized Anxiety Disorder, Depressive Disorder with or without generalized anxiety, versus specific phobia or social anxiety. The HAM-A can thus be used to help further refine formulations of emotional difficulties made by diagnosticians to aid them in formulating many different diagnoses across these commonly co-morbid disorders.

7.2. Monitoring Treatment Progress

If the clinician uses a medication from an evidence-based practice, a dosage sufficient for symptom remission is given for an adequate number of weeks, and the patient symptoms continue, the regimen is adjusted and then re-consolidated. If partial remission of symptoms occurs, adequate augmentation and/or acceleration strategies are used for an adequate amount of time. The treatment can then be deemed unsuccessful, and an alternative medication or psychopharmacological treatment offered for the patient.

The HAM-A can help the clinician decide if the patient being treated has actually responded. Patients who do not demonstrate a clinical response to therapeutic intervention after taking prescribed doses of medication for no less than an adequate amount of time can be considered non-responders. It would be appropriate to make such definitive determinations after trying two occasions of medication increases and/or adding an augmentation or acceleration strategy. Also, it is reasonable to observe both remission and response to medication strategies for 4-6 weeks or longer to ensure efficacy.

Different classes of treatments are currently available for GAD, with various limitations and preferences based on individual patient characteristics, such as comorbid psychiatric disorders or medical conditions. As a result, anxiety often fluctuates, even in the face of a successful treatment. Monitoring treatment progress and the periodic reevaluation of the patient's status could provide the impetus to consider a modification in treatment.

Another major use of a modern anxiety-rating scale is to monitor the progress and outcome of an intervention. This is a valuable way of determining whether a particular treatment is beneficial for the patient and is of extreme clinical importance. It also allows for the modification of treatment as needed. The HAM-A is a sensitive instrument for detecting drug impact, providing a means for measuring a variable that is not easily determined by questioning, making it particularly useful in the assessment of drug treatment.

8. Advantages and Limitations of the Hamilton Anxiety Scale

The Hamilton Anxiety Scale (HAM-A), an 18-item full range modeling tool focusing on anxiety symptoms, is greatly favored. However, it has some limitations. The fact that it is so flexible and open to other updates is a major rate limiting feature of HAM-A. The expert score, often between 3, is reliant on the inter-raters. A strong association with depression has been blamed for the focus it gives on anxiety-related somatic symptoms and its coexisting depression symptoms. Some special knowledge in psychopathology is necessary to use the HAM-A for scientific factors, clinical implications, and recommendations for treatment. Assess the exaggerated symptoms by the separated rating OU to prevent overrating. In general, initial judgments should not be taken at face value and other saucing tools need to be used as well as rated scales.

The Hamilton Anxiety Scale (HAM-A) is complete and easy to administer. The scale covers fewer somatic concerns/issues regarding anxiety, including depression and a few references concerning neurasthenia. Today's HAM-A is most widely used (94% of professionals chose it as the most widely used rating scale used for the clinical rating of anxiety). As well as for testing, it also has idiographic threshold values, making it useful in clinical and further work. Nevertheless, the unnecessary words, genuine distress, and either overvalued or underrated answers raise situations where results cannot be regarded as acceptable.

9. Comparison with Other Anxiety Assessment Tools

The HAM-A, one of the most used and validated scales, should be kept consistent from the transition change from the 1950's version to the 2014 version, whereas it has been steadily changed. The symptom subscale scores, for example, factor analysis as below, have been constantly investigated: psychomotor agitation and somatic muscle effect in the 1950's version; physical anxiety symptoms consisting mainly of muscle symptoms and hyperventilation; nonphysical anxiety subscale consisting of psychomotor agitation and fear in the 1970s and up to the recent 2014 version.

The Hamilton Anxiety Scale (HAM-A) is a well-recognized validated scale used for anxiety assessment among different psychiatric disorders. There are numerous such tools for anxiety assessment, and each tool has its own pros and cons such as simple language, less time-consuming, easy-to-apply, appropriate trigger questions, a combination of different items, better in a specific psychiatric disorder, relevance of chosen items, newer assessment method, and distinguish anxiety from depression. The differentiation of anxiety symptoms from physical illness is quite challenging and it is even more challenging to distinguish these two as separate symptoms. The scores for HAM-A may be variable in nonclinical populations and physical diseases that may be correlated independently with anxiety symptoms or share common symptoms with anxiety that may increase the scores; it is helpful for us to understand the percentage relevance of these symptoms in this specific tool when compared with other anxiety assessments. In comparison with HAM-A-representative data showing finished cases, there are expected results: HAM-A, i.e., 2014 mean for each item among 70 disorders when most of the HAM-A items showed lower than 1.4 as average scores. This study used a Japanese version of the HAM-A 2014 in the general population. Additionally, HAM-A is still the most valid tool to be used in the study and treatment trial.

10. Use of the Scale in Research Studies

Researchers often employ scales that focus on clinical criteria (i.e., Diagnostic and Statistical Manual IIIR or IV or a particular ICD version) to help provide evidence of a dose-response relationship between a drug and the disease being treated. While there is some merit to this approach, due to the possibility of capturing the so-called "false positive," the utilization of the criteria-focused scales may result in a failure to detect beneficial effects of a drug on anxiety that fall outside of, or extend beyond those described in a specific diagnostic, cross-walking manual. Indeed, this issue extends not only to the efficacious drugs themselves (e.g., alprazolam and buspirone, which failed to show efficacy when analyzed with the Food and Drug Administration's, or FDA's notion of what an outcome research tool should be) but is applicable in a significant number of prescriptions that are written in the United States. Per typical pharmaceutical marketing data, more than 50 percent of anxiolytics are currently being prescribed for a diagnosis of anxiety, in which no DSM clinical disorder is labeled for escalation to prescription status. Thus, there is a large, unmet and under-recognized demand for mood and anxiety disorder or symptom-based scientific inquiry, which can in turn justify intellectual property for those manufacturers who research that product with such scales.

The utilization of the Hamilton Anxiety Scale (HAM-A) in research studies has become widespread. The HAM-A frequently serves as a research instrument when the main focus of an investigation is not on the assessment of anxiety, but rather on a related disease state or an investigation of other related processes. The HAM-A has been incorporated into research in a number of areas. First, the HAM-A has been employed in studies that are investigating the relationship of specific pathologies with comorbid or syndromal anxiety, including Attention Deficit/Hyperactivity Disorder, Inflammatory Bowel Disease, and endometriosis. It has also been used to measure the primary efficacy of, or as an outcome measure in, drug studies in diverse areas such as Antisocial personality, Alzheimer's Disease, Bipolar Disorder, Major Depressive Disorder, Multiple Sclerosis, Schizophrenia, Post Traumatic Stress Disorder, and shyness. In addition to these areas, the HAM-A has been chosen and validated as a research instrument in studies of anxiety. The elements underlying the HAM-A that make it of special value for this use are discussed below.

11. Self-Administered Versions of the Scale

A few alternative versions of the HAM-A scale (aside from the self-administered version) have been forwarded, also to limit the burden on patients and raters. Four items shown in a previous Korean RCT of escitalopram to have the highest sensitivity to change in severity of anxiety have been put forward for use as a 'core' 4-item anxiety subscale as an abbreviated, self-rating tool drawing on this work. There have been two questions as to how this abbreviated rating subscale relates to the longer HAM-A form that might also be posed with self-administered versions.

Given significant advances in the development of web-based platforms and electronic interfaces, it has been suggested that HAM-A and other observer-administered assessment tools could have self-administered counterparts. Self-administered tools have both strong advantages and limitations. Because patients can use them unaided, self-administered tools greatly increase the accessibility of assessment and can easily be administered on a larger scale. They also have particular value in research settings, where they can provide quick, easy, and relatively inexpensive-to-collect data for subjects who might be participating in a trial from different geographic areas or patient populations. On the other hand, there is often some concern that patients might misunderstand the questions or miss the subtlety of the emotional assessments that are solicited in a structured interview.

Studies that have compared self-administered versions of rating scales with structured interviews have shown they are typically lower in rigor than the interviewer-administered versions and produce inflated responses. The most important question, however, would be if self-administered versions would be acceptable to drug development regulators who favor 'hard' measures of disease activity.

The HAM-A has been administered via electronic tablets, Facsimile-Back Data Entry (FDE) and Interactive Voice Recognition (IVR) technologies, by mail, and, most commonly, by paper and pencil. The primary advantage of modes other than paper and pencil comes in terms of data management. Electronic tablets allow instant availability of self-administered HAM-A data in digital format, while Facsimile-Back Data Entry was used specifically to collect digital HAM-A data in areas without Internet connections. IVR systems are suitable for large population-based studies, although participants with severe symptoms may have trouble listening to instructions or manipulating number keys. The Hamilton Anxiety Scale was originally developed to be used by clinicians, involving direct dialogue between the administrator (usually a physician) and the patient. Most patients in the studies involving the HAM-A self-rated it in the absence of direct contact with a health care worker. Management of the clinical information of participants who self-assess with the HAM-A (whether on tablets, smartphones, or consignment of postal questionnaires) must therefore depend on the study design, existing resources, and infrastructure for managing self-information of other kinds. These practicalities, in turn, define whether HAM-A data can be retrieved from electronic devices by direct download or require data entry, and prompt decisions about the governance and ethics of data management, in relation to data protection legislation and local research protocols. The feasibility of different forms of data retrieval was not tested in this study. Compliance is also strongly related to the participant level of distress, which affects engagement with research protocols in general. Only one study has compared the HAM-A scores from two different modes of self-administration. In this study, 71 individuals completed the HAM-A as part of a psychiatric consultation and also completed it again at home.

The HAM-A has been translated into 37 languages for self-administered use, and large population-based studies have employed it in this way, including the NESDA cohort. The feasibility of large-scale self-administered HAM-A administration is reflected in our study sample of 11,414 individuals. From a practical perspective, self-administration is appealing because of its potential for significant time-savings and, arguably of equal importance in the current climate, reduces the need for patients to interact with clinicians, decreasing the likelihood of nosocomial COVID-19 infections. However, the HAM-A is a clinical instrument and, unlike self-administered scales designed for use first in research settings, it was not initially created to be self-administered. Research-level scales are specifically validated for self-administration and reliability, validity, and practical utility need to be re-assessed when the mode of administration is changed from clinician-administered to self-administered. Furthermore, the HAM-A does not lend itself to the parallel self-administered/clinician-administered validation approaches used for comparison.

12. Resources for Accessing the Hamilton Anxiety Scale

ResearchGate offers a discussion and download of a version of the Hamilton Anxiety Scale: "Anxiety has been conceptualized as an interfering and impairing antecedent or crucial component of various problems (i.e. fear, phobia, stress, depression, negative affect, rumination, avoidance, dysfunctional behavior, low-quality of life, reduced interpersonal effectiveness, academic performance). Thus, a rising interest for an item (i.e., anxiety) that makes a difference, has gone somewhat unnoticed in the overwhelming task of treatment and assessment. 1504 Madison, WI: American Professional Credentialing Services." Further information may be obtained from.

It is possible to purchase and download the complete Hamilton Anxiety Scale and accompanying instructions, item by item. A description of the Hamilton Anxiety Scale, sample reports, and the option for purchasing the scale with complete instructions can be found at.

There are several resources that contain the Hamilton Anxiety Scale (HAM-A) in their entirety, together with permission to reproduce instructions for clients or subjects when using the scale. The first of these resources is the oft-cited reference article for the scale by Hamilton, which has been reproduced in full earlier in this collection. An additional excellent and cost-effective resource for obtaining the HAM-A is found at Clinical Psychology

Resources. The inventory that is included is "Hamilton Anxiety Rating Scale - Iowa Version 1 (HAM-A), available in both a convenient hard-copy format ($10) and a hard-copy/CD-ROM format ($30)."

EL FESTÍN DE LOS MEDIOCRES

Reflexiones sobre el fanatismo, la mezquindad y la ignorancia

Dr. Javier González Maciel

DEDICATORIA

A mi amada hija María con el amor eterno de su padre